Menopause diet plan book

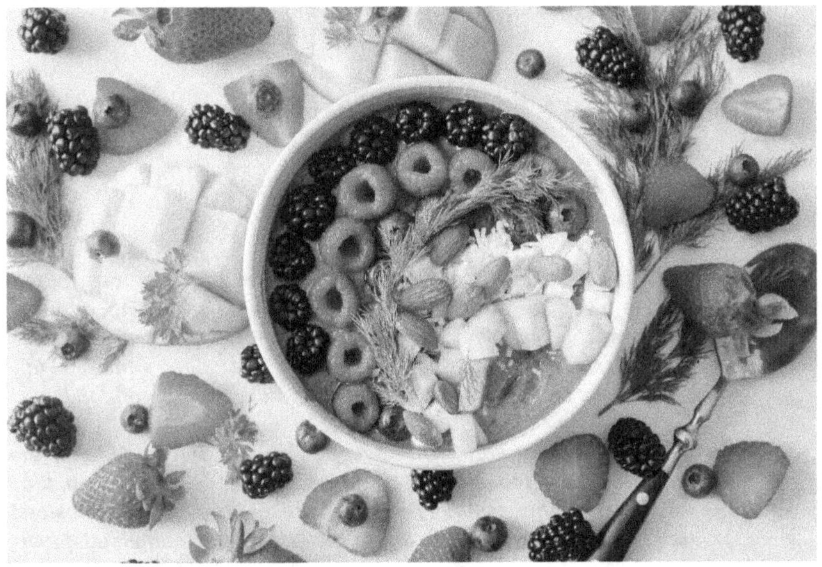

A guide to stay young, and healthy and manage Hormones

SANTA G HOOPER

Table of content

Table of content
Introduction
CHAPTER ONE
    Reasons why you need menopause diet plan
CHAPTER TWO
    Consider taking your health to heart
CHAPTER THREE
    Reducing the risk of diabetes
CHAPTER FOUR
    Brain protection
CHAPTER FIVE
    Reducing the risk of cancer
CHAPTER SIX
    Dietary Supplements that helps before and after Menopause
CHAPTER SEVEN
    The menopause diet plan
        Breakfast:
        Mid-Morning Snack:
        Afternoon Snack:
        Evening Snack (if needed):
CHAPTER EIGHT
    Healthy Eating Tips For Menopause
CONCLUSION

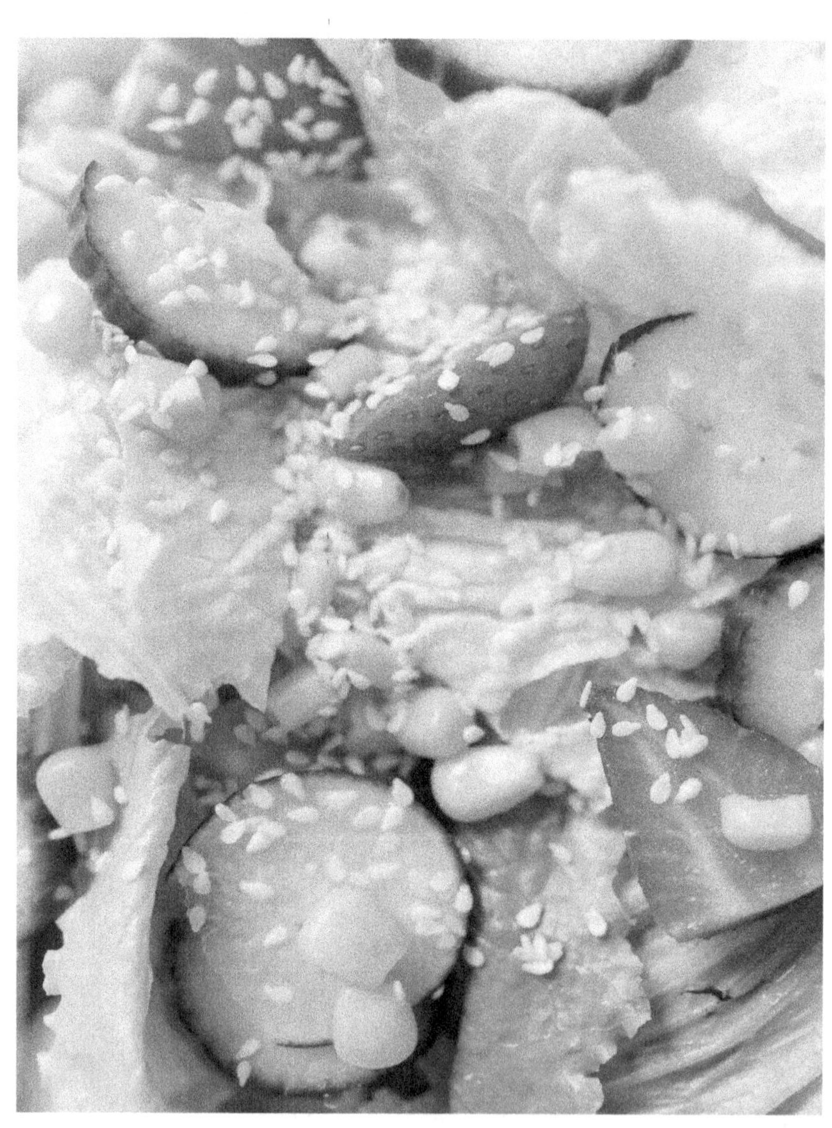

Introduction

Welcome to "The Menopause Diet Plan," a comprehensive guide designed to empower women as they navigate the transformative phase of menopause. This book is your key to understanding the profound impact of diet on your overall well-being during this crucial stage of life.

Menopause is a natural birth process that every woman experiences as she reaches the mid-period. It marks the end of reproductive capabilities, accompanied by significant hormonal changes. These changes can bring about various physical and emotional challenges, including hot flashes, mood swings, weight gain, and increased risk of chronic diseases.

However, the good news is that with the right knowledge and a well-structured diet plan, women can not only manage the symptoms of menopause but also enjoy vibrant health, vitality, and a sense of youthfulness throughout this life transition.

In "The Menopause Diet Plan," we will explore:

Understanding Menopause: We'll delve into the science behind menopause, explaining the hormonal shifts and their effects on your body and mind. This knowledge will serve as the foundation for your journey toward better health.

The Role of Diet: Discover how the foods you eat directly impact your hormonal balance, metabolism, and overall health during menopause. Learn which nutrients are essential and how to incorporate them into your daily meals.

Hormone Management: Explore natural ways to manage hormones without resorting to medication. We'll discuss how diet can influence estrogen levels, alleviate mood swings, and reduce the severity of hot flashes.

Weight Management: Menopause often brings weight gain, but we'll provide you with strategies to maintain a healthy weight through nutrition and exercise tailored specifically to your needs.

Bone Health: Understand the significance of bone health during menopause and learn how to protect your bones through diet and lifestyle choices.

Heart Health: Discover dietary habits that promote cardiovascular well-being, reducing the risk of heart disease, which can increase after menopause.

Emotional Well-being: Explore the connection between nutrition and mood, and how a well-balanced diet can help you maintain a positive outlook during this life stage.

Recipes and Meal Plans: Find delicious and nutritious recipes designed to support your hormonal balance and overall health. We've included customizable meal plans to make your transition to a menopause-friendly diet seamless.

Lifestyle Tips: Beyond diet, we'll provide advice on lifestyle adjustments, including stress management, exercise, and sleep, to ensure you thrive during menopause.

"The Menopause Diet Plan" is not just a book; it's your trusted companion on your journey to renewed vitality, health, and a profound understanding of how the choices you make today can shape your future. Whether you're experiencing the early signs of menopause or are well into this phase, this book will empower you to take control of your health and embrace the wisdom and strength that come with this new chapter of life. Get ready to embrace menopause with confidence and grace, and discover how to stay young, healthy, and hormonally balanced.

CHAPTER ONE

Reasons why you need menopause diet plan

A menopause diet plan is essential for women going through this life stage for several reasons:

Hormonal Changes: Menopause marks the end of a woman's reproductive years and brings about significant hormonal fluctuations, including a decrease in estrogen levels. These hormonal changes can lead to various symptoms, such as hot flashes, mood swings, and weight gain.

Weight Management: Many women experience weight gain during menopause due to a slower metabolism and changes in body composition. A well-designed diet plan can help manage weight and prevent obesity-related health issues, such as heart disease and diabetes.

Bone Health Estrogen plays a critical part in maintaining bone thickness. With lower estrogen levels during menopause, women are at a higher risk of osteoporosis and fractures. A menopause diet rich in calcium and vitamin D can help support bone health.

Heart Health: Estrogen also has a protective effect on the cardiovascular system. As estrogen levels decline, the risk of heart disease increases. A heart-healthy diet plan can help reduce the risk of heart-related issues.

Mood and Mental Health: Hormonal changes during menopause can lead to mood swings, anxiety, and depression. Nutrient-rich foods can have a positive impact on mood and mental well-being by providing essential vitamins and minerals.

Digestive Health: Some women experience digestive problems during menopause, such as bloating and constipation. A diet plan that includes fiber-rich foods can aid in maintaining good digestive health.

Hot Flashes and Night Sweats: Certain foods and beverages, like caffeine, alcohol, and spicy foods, can trigger hot flashes and night sweats. A menopause diet plan can help identify and avoid these triggers.

Energy Levels: Fatigue and decreased energy are common complaints during menopause. A balanced diet that includes complex carbohydrates and protein can help stabilize energy levels.

Hormone Balance: Specific foods contain phytoestrogens, which are plant compounds that mimic the effects of estrogen in the body. Incorporating these foods into a menopausal diet can help support hormone balance.

Long-Term Health: Menopause is a transitional period, but it also marks the beginning of a new phase of life. A well-planned menopause diet can establish healthy eating habits that contribute to overall health and well-being in the post-menopausal years.

In summary, a menopause diet plan is essential because it addresses the unique challenges and health risks associated with this life stage. By focusing on nutrition tailored to menopausal needs, women can better manage symptoms, support their long-term health, and improve their overall quality of life during and after menopause.

CHAPTER TWO

Consider taking your health to heart

Taking Your Health to Heart" emphasizes the critical role that nutrition plays in heart health during and after menopause. Menopause is a time of significant hormonal changes, particularly a decline in estrogen levels. These hormonal shifts can have a direct impact on cardiovascular health, making it essential for women to proactively manage their heart health through dietary choices. Here's a comprehensive look at how to take your health to heart with a menopause diet plan:

. Understand the Cardiovascular Risks: Women going through menopause face an increased risk of heart disease. This is partly because estrogen, which has a protective effect on the cardiovascular system, decreases. It's crucial to recognize these heightened risks and take proactive steps to mitigate them.

. Prioritize Heart-Healthy Nutrients: Your menopause diet plan should prioritize foods rich in heart-healthy nutrients. These include:

- Omega-3 Fatty Acids: Found in fatty fish like salmon and walnuts, these fats can help reduce inflammation and lower the risk of heart disease.
- Fiber: Foods high in soluble fiber like oats, beans, and fruits can help lower cholesterol levels and maintain a healthy weight.
- Antioxidants: Berries, leafy greens, and other colorful fruits and vegetables are rich in antioxidants that protect the heart from damage.
- Whole Grains: Opt for whole grains like quinoa, brown rice, and whole wheat, which provide sustained energy and support heart health.

.Control Cholesterol Levels: Menopausal women should be especially vigilant about their cholesterol levels. A diet low in saturated fats and trans fats while high in soluble fiber can help maintain healthy cholesterol levels.

.Monitor Blood Pressure: High blood pressure is a risk factor for heart disease. A diet low in sodium (salt) and high in potassium, found in foods like bananas, sweet potatoes, and spinach, can help regulate blood pressure.

.Limit Added Sugars and Processed Foods: Excessive sugar intake and highly processed foods can contribute to weight gain and increase the risk of heart disease. Avoid sugary drinks, candies, and heavily processed snacks.

.Stay Hydrated: Proper hydration is required for heart health. Aim to drink plenty of water throughout the day and limit sticky drinks.

.Manage Weight: Many women experience weight gain during menopause. A balanced diet that aligns with your caloric needs can help maintain a healthy weight, reducing the risk of heart disease.

.Exercise Regularly: Complement your menopause diet plan with regular physical activity. Exercise helps maintain a healthy weight, lowers blood pressure, and strengthens the heart muscle.

.Consult a Healthcare Provider: It's crucial to consult with your healthcare provider or a registered dietitian to create a personalized menopause diet plan that addresses your specific health needs, including any existing medical conditions or medications.

.Lifestyle Factors: Alongside nutrition, managing stress, getting enough sleep, and avoiding smoking are vital components of heart health. Incorporating stress-reduction techniques like meditation or yoga into your routine can be beneficial.

In conclusion, taking your health to heart during menopause involves a holistic approach to nutrition and lifestyle choices. A well-structured menopause diet plan that prioritizes heart-healthy foods, along with regular exercise and overall self-care, can significantly reduce the risk of heart disease and promote overall well-being during this life stage. Consulting with healthcare professionals is crucial to tailor a plan that suits your individual needs and helps you navigate the challenges of menopause while safeguarding your heart health.

CHAPTER THREE

Reducing the risk of diabetes

Reducing the risk of diabetes is crucial, especially considering the rising prevalence of this chronic condition worldwide. Both Type 1 diabetes (an autoimmune condition) and Type 2 diabetes (usually associated with lifestyle factors) benefit from risk reduction strategies. Here's a comprehensive overview of how to reduce the risk of diabetes:

1. Redundant body weight, especially around the tummy, increases the threat of Type 2 diabetes.

Aim for a balanced diet and regular physical exercise to achieve and maintain a healthy weight.

Losing even a modest amount of weight (5-10% of your current weight) can significantly reduce diabetes risk.

2. Adopt a Balanced Diet:

Focus on a diet rich in whole grains, thin proteins, healthy fats, and a variety of fruits and vegetables.

Choose water, herbal tea, or tart potables rather.

Control portion sizes to manage calorie intake.

3. Monitor Carbohydrate Intake:

Be conscious of the kind and quantity of carbohydrates you consume.

Choose complex carbohydrates (e.g., whole grains, legumes) over simple sugars (e.g., candy, sugary drinks).

Be mindful of portion sizes to avoid spikes in blood sugar levels.

4. Increase Fiber Intake:

Fiber-rich foods like whole grains, fruits, vegetables, and legumes help stabilize blood sugar levels and improve insulin sensitivity.

5. Limit Sugary Beverages:

Sugary drinks are a major contributor to diabetes risk. Consider water, herbal tea, or unsweetened drinks instead.

6. Watch Your Fat Intake:

Opt for healthy fats such as those found in avocados, nuts, seeds, and fatty fish.

Reduce permeated and induced fats seen in fried meals and processed snacks.

7. Be Physically Active:

Regular exercise improves insulin sensitivity and helps maintain a healthy weight.

Aim for at least 150 minutes of moderate-intensity aerobic activity or 75 minutes of vigorous-intensity activity per week.

8. Strength Training:

Include strength training exercises at least two days a week to build muscle, which can aid in blood sugar control.

9. Manage Stress:

Chronic stress can raise blood sugar levels. Practice stress-reduction approaches like awareness, contemplation, or yoga.

10. Get Quality Sleep:

Poor sleep patterns may contribute to insulin resistance. Aspire for 7-9 hours of quality sleep every night.

11. Limit Alcohol Consumption: If you choose to drink alcohol, do so in temperance

Limit to one drink per day for women and two drinks per day for men.

12. Regular Check-ups:

Visit your healthcare provider regularly for routine check-ups and diabetes screenings, especially if you have risk factors like a family history of diabetes or obesity.

13. Avoid Smoking:

Smoking is associated with an increased threat of Type 2 diabetes. Seek support to quit if you are a smoker.

14. Know Your Family History:

A family record of diabetes can increase your risk. Be knowledgeable of your family's health history and talk with your healthcare provider.

15. Stay Informed:

Continuously educate yourself about diabetes risk factors, prevention, and management.

Remember that reducing the risk of diabetes is a lifelong commitment. It involves making sustainable lifestyle changes that promote overall health and well-being. Consulting with a healthcare professional or registered dietitian can provide personalized guidance and support on your journey to lower diabetes risk.

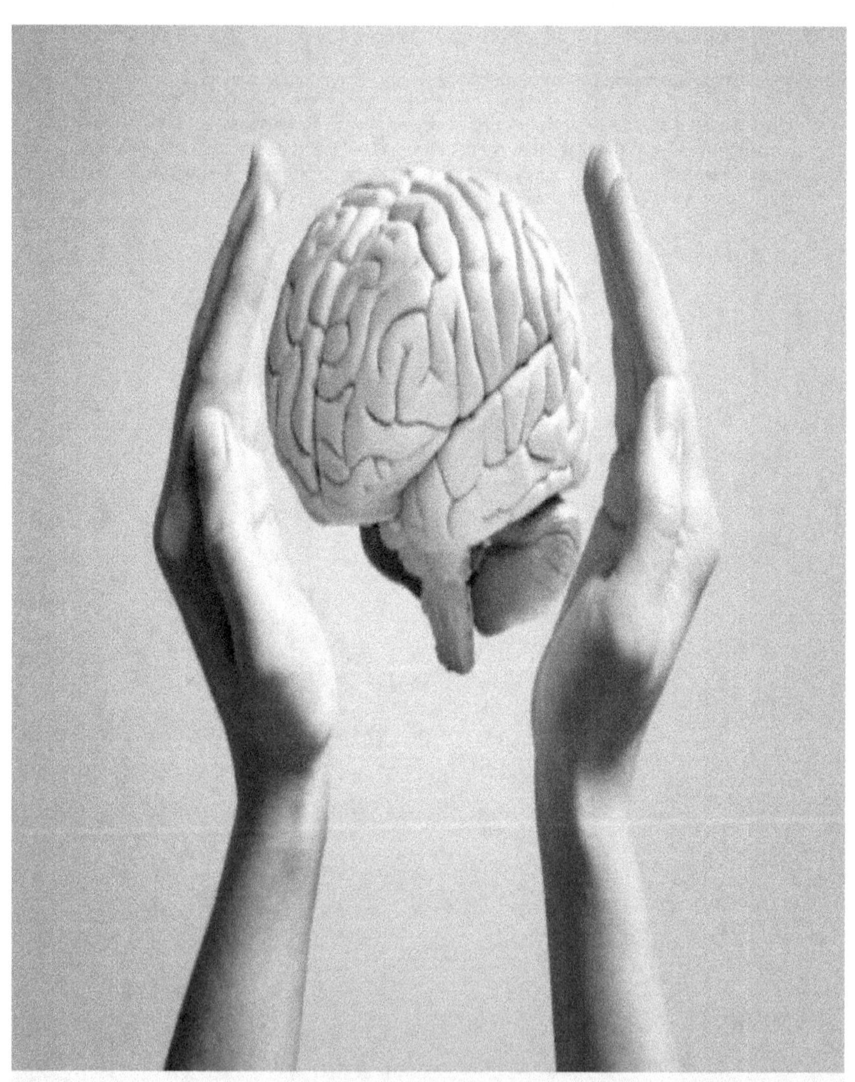

CHAPTER FOUR

Brain protection

Protecting your brain during and after menopause is crucial for maintaining cognitive function, emotional well-being, and overall quality of life. Hormonal changes during menopause can affect brain health, but there are strategies you can adopt to protect your brain. Here's a comprehensive guide:

Hormone Replacement Therapy (HRT):

Talk with a professional healthcare provider about the probable benefits and dangers of HRT. HRT may help alleviate some menopausal symptoms and support brain health in certain cases.

A Balanced Diet:

Eat a brain-healthy diet rich in fruits, vegetables, whole grains, lean proteins, and healthy fats.

Omega-3 fatty acids found in fatty fish (e.g., salmon), flaxseeds, and walnuts are particularly beneficial for brain health.

Manage Blood Sugar Levels:

Maintaining steady blood sugar levels by eating up complex carbohydrates and evading extreme sugar intake.

High blood sugar can sum up cognitive deterioration.

Stay Hydrated:

Dehydration can affect cognitive function. Take a surplus intake of water throughout the day.

Regular Exercise:

Engage in regular physical activity, which improves blood flow to the brain and supports cognitive function.

Cardiovascular activity and strength exercises are helpful.

Mental Stimulation:

Maintain your active brain with puzzles, games, reading, or learning new skills.

Social interaction and engaging in meaningful conversations also stimulate cognitive function.

Adequate Sleep:

Prioritize good sleep to let your brain rest and converge memories.

Address sleep disturbances common during menopause, such as night sweats or insomnia.

Stress Management:

Chronic stress can negatively impact brain health. Practice stress-reduction procedures like reflection, mindfulness, or yoga.

Hormone Balance:

Consult with your healthcare provider about hormone balance during menopause. Hormonal fluctuations can affect mood and cognitive function.

Manage Mood and Emotions:

Mood swings and emotional changes are common during menopause. Strive for help from a therapist or counselor if required.

Consider mindfulness and relaxation techniques to manage emotions.

Heart Health:

What's satisfactory for your heart is usually good for your brain. Manage cardiovascular risk factors by eating a heart-healthy diet and exercising regularly.

Regular Health Check-ups:

Stay proactive about your health with regular check-ups. Discuss any cognitive concerns or memory changes with your healthcare provider.

Bone Health:

Osteoporosis can increase the risk of falls and head injuries. Maintain strong bones through a diet rich in calcium and vitamin D and regular weight-bearing exercise.

Hormone Health:

Talk to your healthcare provider about the impact of hormonal changes on brain health.

Explore alternative therapies such as acupuncture or herbal remedies if they align with your healthcare plan.

Medication Review:

Review your medications with your healthcare provider, as some drugs may affect cognitive function.

Avoid Smoking and Limit Alcohol:

Smoking and exorbitant alcohol intake can cause harm to your brain's health. Stop smoking if you smoke and drink alcohol with restraint.

Community Engagement:

Stay socially active and engaged with your community to combat feelings of isolation and loneliness.

Stay Informed:

Keep up-to-date with the latest research on menopause and brain health to make informed choices.

Remember that brain health is a lifelong journey, and adopting these strategies can benefit women not only during menopause but also throughout their lives. If you notice significant cognitive changes or memory problems, consult a healthcare professional for a comprehensive evaluation and guidance tailored to your specific needs.

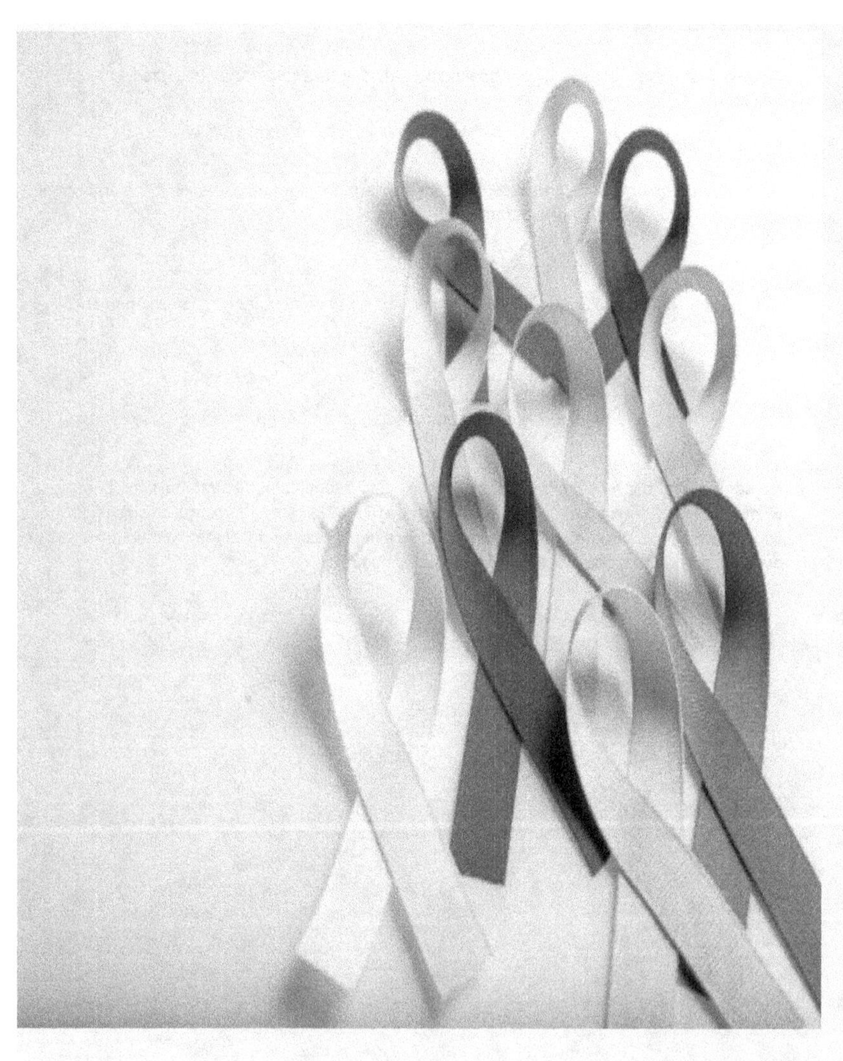

CHAPTER FIVE

Reducing the risk of cancer

Reducing the risk of cancer, including breast and ovarian cancer, is a significant concern for many women during and after menopause. While diet alone cannot guarantee cancer prevention, it can play a substantial role in reducing your risk. Here are some dietary procedures to contemplate:

.Eat a Plant-Based Diet:

- Focus on a diet rich in fruits, vegetables, whole grains, legumes, and nuts.
- These foods are packed with antioxidants and phytochemicals that can help protect against cancer.

. Colorful Fruits and Vegetables:

- Consume a variety of colorful fruits and vegetables, as different colors indicate different cancer-fighting compounds.
- Tomatoes, berries, broccoli, kale, and carrots are particularly beneficial.

. Limit Red and Processed Meats:

- High consumption of red and processed meats is associated with an increased risk of several cancers.
- Opt for thin protein bases like poultry, fish, beans, and tofu.

. Choose Healthy Fats:

- Use olive oil or canola oil instead of saturated or trans fats found in fried foods and processed snacks.
- Omega-3 fatty acids from sources like fatty fish (e.g., salmon) can be protective against some types of cancer.

. Reduce Sugar and Processed Foods:

- High sugar intake and processed foods may contribute to obesity, which is a risk factor for several cancers.
- Minimize sugary drinks, snacks, and foods with added sugars.

. Limit Alcohol Intake:

- Excessive alcohol consumption is linked to an increased risk of breast and other cancers.

- If you drink alcohol, do so in moderation (one drink per day for women).

. Increase Fiber Intake:

- Foods high in fiber, such as whole grains, legumes, and vegetables, can help reduce the risk of colorectal cancer.

. Calcium and Vitamin D:

- Adequate calcium and vitamin D intake is important for maintaining bone health and may reduce the risk of certain cancers.
- Dairy foods, fortified foods, and supplements can enable satisfy these needs.

. Cruciferous Vegetables:

- Have cruciferous vegetables like broccoli, cauliflower, and Brussels nodes in your diet.
- They contain compounds that may help protect against cancer.

. Stay Hydrated:

- Gulp plenty of water throughout the day to sustain general health.

. Limit Processed and Canned Foods:

- Processed and canned foods often contain preservatives and additives that may have cancer-related risks.
- Opt for fresh or frozen alternatives.

. Moderate Caffeine Intake:

- Some studies suggest that excessive caffeine consumption may increase the risk of certain cancers.
- Limit your caffeine intake, particularly from sugary or artificially flavored beverages.

. Mindful Eating:

- Pay attention to portion sizes and avoid overeating, which can contribute to weight gain.

. Stay Informed:

- Stay informed about the latest research on diet and cancer prevention, as new findings can impact dietary recommendations.

. Consult a Dietitian:

- Consider consulting a registered dietitian who can provide personalized dietary guidance based on your specific needs and risk factors.

It's important to note that while a healthy diet can reduce cancer risk, it should be combined with other preventive measures such as regular screenings, maintaining a healthy weight, staying physically active, and avoiding tobacco products. Additionally, individual risk factors and genetic predispositions play a role in cancer development, so it's essential to discuss your risk and preventive strategies with your healthcare provider.

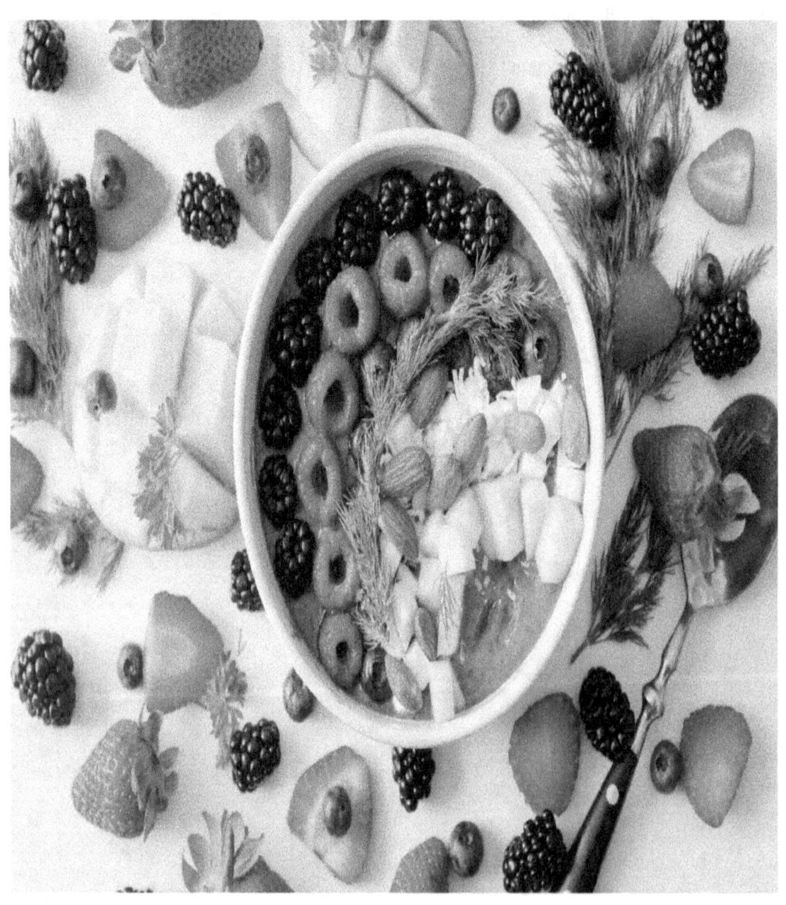

CHAPTER SIX

Dietary Supplements that helps before and after Menopause

Dietary supplements can be beneficial before and during menopause to help manage symptoms and support overall health. However, it's important to consult with a healthcare provider or registered dietitian before starting any new supplements, as individual needs and potential interactions with medications can vary. Here are some dietary supplements that are commonly considered during menopause:

. Calcium and Vitamin D:

- These are essential for maintaining bone health. Menopausal women are at an increased risk of osteoporosis, so adequate calcium (usually around 1,200-1,500 mg daily) and vitamin D (often 600-800 IU daily) intake is important.

. Magnesium:

- Magnesium supports bone health and may help alleviate symptoms like insomnia, anxiety, and muscle cramps.

. Vitamin K:

- Vitamin K is involved in bone health and may help with calcium absorption. It's often found in leafy greens and can be supplemented if necessary.

. Omega-3 Fatty Acids:

- These can aid in decreasing inflammation and support cardiovascular health. They are found in fish oil supplements.

. Black Cohosh:

- Black cohosh is a popular herbal supplement for relieving hot flashes and mood swings during menopause. It may have estrogen-like effects.

. Soy Isoflavones:

- Soy isoflavones contain phytoestrogens, which may help alleviate menopausal symptoms. They are available in supplement form but are also found in foods like tofu and soybeans.

. Evening Primrose Oil:

- Some women use evening primrose oil to relieve symptoms like breast tenderness and mood swings.

. Red Clover:

- Red clover is another source of phytoestrogens and is used by some women to manage menopausal symptoms.

. Vitamin E:

- Vitamin E supplements may help alleviate hot flashes and night sweats in some women.

. Probiotics:

- Probiotic supplements can promote digestive health and help with any gastrointestinal issues that may arise during menopause.

. Iron (if needed):

- Iron supplements may be necessary for women with iron-deficiency anemia.

. B Vitamins:

- B vitamins, particularly B6 and B12, can help with mood swings and overall energy levels.

. Melatonin:

- Melatonin supplements may aid in improving sleep quality, which can be disrupted during menopause.

. Maca Root:

- Some women use maca root supplements to boost energy and alleviate menopausal symptoms.

. Multivitamin:

- A good quality multivitamin can assist in filling in nutritional voids in your diet.

Recall that supplements should not be a stand-in for a balanced diet. Whenever possible, try to obtain essential nutrients from whole foods. Additionally, supplements should be taken as recommended, and it's important not to exceed the recommended doses, as excessive intake can have adverse effects.

Before taking any dietary supplements during menopause, consult with your healthcare provider or a registered dietitian. They can assess your specific needs, consider potential interactions with medications, and provide personalized guidance to help you manage menopausal symptoms and support your overall health.

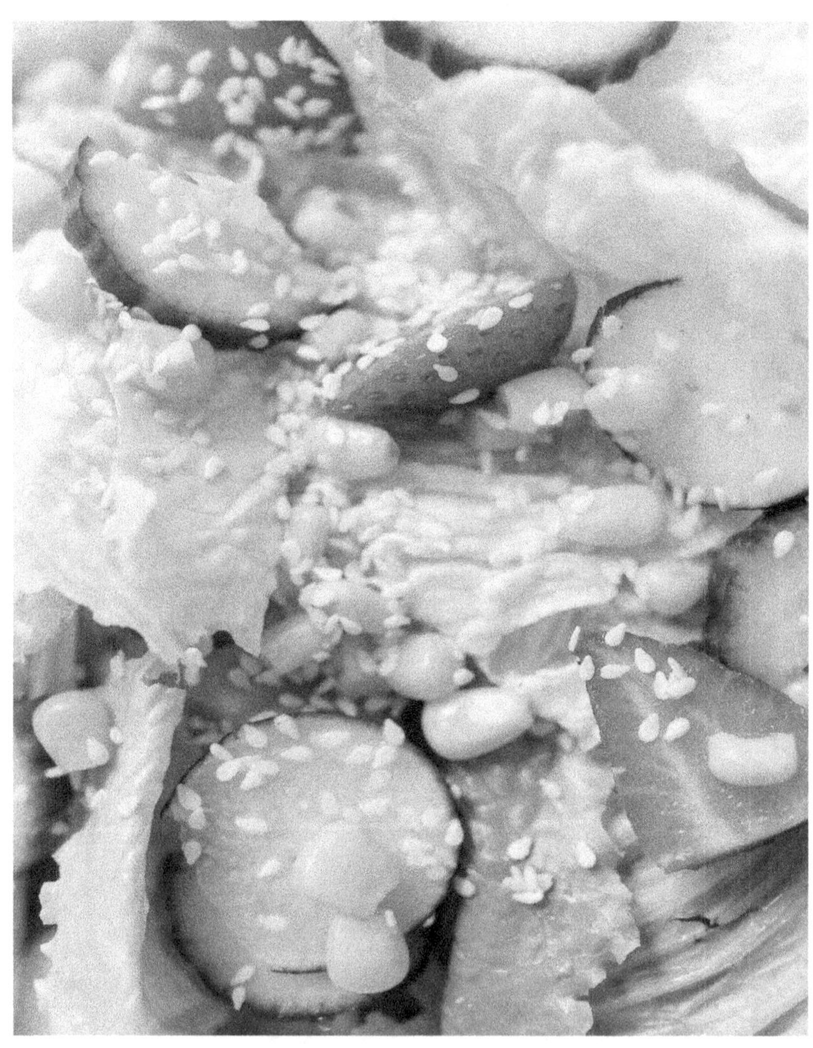

CHAPTER SEVEN

The menopause diet plan

A well-balanced menopause diet plan focuses on addressing the unique nutritional needs of women going through this life stage while managing symptoms and supporting overall health. Here's a detailed menopause diet plan:

Breakfast:

. Whole-Grain Cereal: Start your day with a bowl of whole-grain cereal (e.g., oatmeal or bran flakes) topped with fresh berries (antioxidants) and a sprinkle of flaxseeds (omega-3 fatty acids and fiber).

. Greek Yogurt: Include a serving of Greek yogurt for calcium and protein.

. Green Tea: Sip on green tea, which may help with weight management and hot flashes.

Mid-Morning Snack:

. Mixed Nuts: Enjoy a small handful of mixed nuts (e.g., almonds, walnuts) for healthy fats and satiety.

Lunch:

. Salad: Have a large salad with leafy greens, colorful vegetables, and lean protein like grilled chicken or tofu.

. Quinoa: Add a side of quinoa or brown rice for fiber and nutrients.

. Olive Oil Dressing: Use olive oil and balsamic vinegar as dressing for healthy fats.

Afternoon Snack:

. Carrot Sticks with Hummus: Munch on carrot sticks dipped in hummus for a satisfying and nutritious snack.

Dinner:

. Grilled Salmon: Enjoy a serving of grilled salmon, a great source of omega-3 fatty acids.

. Steamed Broccoli: Serve steamed broccoli or other cruciferous vegetables for added fiber and antioxidants.

. Sweet Potato: Include a sweet potato for complex carbohydrates and beta-carotene.

Evening Snack (if needed):

. Low-Fat Cottage Cheese: Opt for a small serving of low-fat cottage cheese for protein and calcium.

Beverages:

. Water: Be hydrated all through the day by consuming an abundance of water.

. Herbal Tea: Consider herbal teas like chamomile or peppermint for relaxation in the evening.

Notes:

- Portion Control: Pay attention to portion sizes to manage calorie intake and prevent weight gain, a common issue during menopause.
- Calcium: Ensure you meet your daily calcium needs (around 1,200-1,500 mg) through dairy products, fortified foods, or supplements if necessary.
- Omega-3 Fatty Acids: Consume fatty fish (salmon, mackerel) at least twice a week for omega-3s, or consider fish oil supplements.
- Fiber: Aim for at least 25 grams of fiber daily to support digestive health and manage weight.
- Limit Processed Foods: Minimize processed foods, sugary snacks, and high-sodium items to reduce the risk of heart-related issues.
- Limit Alcohol: If you consume alcohol, do so with restraint (one drink per day for women).
- Nutrient-Dense Choices: Focus on nutrient-dense foods like fruits, vegetables, whole grains, lean proteins, and healthy fats.
- Variety: Have a different variety of foods to provide you with a wide range of nutrients.
- Regular Exercise: Combine this diet plan with regular physical activity, including both cardiovascular exercise and strength training, for the best results.

Remember that this is a general menopause diet plan. Individual nutritional needs can vary based on factors like age, activity level, and any existing health conditions. Consulting with a registered dietitian or healthcare provider can provide personalized guidance and ensure that you're meeting your specific dietary needs during menopause.

CHAPTER EIGHT

Healthy Eating Tips For Menopause

A well-planned menopause diet and following healthy eating tips can help women navigate this life stage with greater ease, manage symptoms, and support overall health. Here's a comprehensive guide to creating and incorporating smart eating habits:

. Control Portion Sizes:

- Pay attention to portion sizes to avoid overeating and manage calorie intake.

. Regular Meals:

- Eat regular meals and snacks to stabilize blood sugar levels and reduce the likelihood of overindulging.

. Mindful Eating:

- Eat slowly and savor each bite. This can help with digestion and prevent overeating.

. Stay Active:

- Regular physical activity helps with weight management and overall health during menopause.

. Stress Management:

- Practice stress-reduction techniques like meditation, deep breathing, or yoga to alleviate emotional eating.

. Monitor Alcohol and Caffeine:

- Be mindful of alcohol and caffeine intake, as they can trigger hot flashes and impact sleep.

. Stay Hydrated:

- Drink water regularly, especially if you're experiencing night sweats.

. Seek Professional Guidance:

- Consult with a registered dietitian or healthcare provider for personalized dietary recommendations and to address specific menopausal symptoms.

Remember that menopause is a unique experience for every woman, and dietary needs may vary. By following a balanced menopause diet plan and adopting healthy eating habits, you can better manage symptoms and support your overall health during this transitional period.

CONCLUSION

In conclusion, a well-structured menopause diet plan and the adoption of healthy eating habits can be transformative during this pivotal phase of life. By nourishing your body with nutrient-rich foods, staying hydrated, controlling portion sizes, and managing stress, you can empower yourself to manage menopausal symptoms effectively and safeguard your long-term health.

Remember, your journey through menopause is unique, and what works best for you may differ from others. Seek guidance from healthcare professionals or registered dietitians to tailor your diet plan to your specific needs, taking into account factors like age, activity level, and any existing health conditions.

Embrace this opportunity to prioritize your well-being through mindful nutrition, and you'll discover that a balanced menopause diet plan is not just about managing symptoms; it's about embracing a healthier, more vibrant, and fulfilling phase of life. Your diet can be your ally in navigating this transition with grace and vitality, supporting you every step of the way toward a healthier, happier menopause journey.